YOUR KNOWLEDGE HAS VALUE

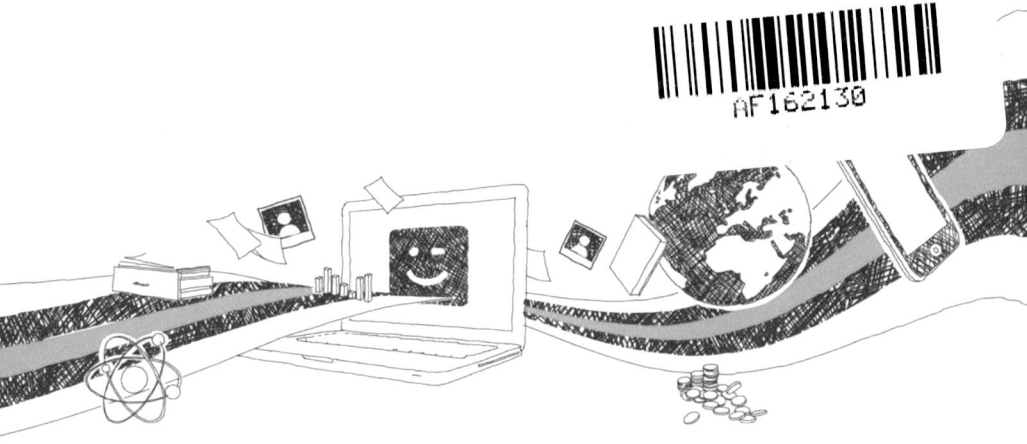

- We will publish your bachelor's and
  master's thesis, essays and papers

- Your own eBook and book -
  sold worldwide in all relevant shops

- Earn money with each sale

Upload your text at www.GRIN.com
and publish for free

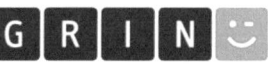

Bibliographic information published by the German National Library:

The German National Library lists this publication in the National Bibliography; detailed bibliographic data are available on the Internet at http://dnb.dnb.de .

This book is copyright material and must not be copied, reproduced, transferred, distributed, leased, licensed or publicly performed or used in any way except as specifically permitted in writing by the publishers, as allowed under the terms and conditions under which it was purchased or as strictly permitted by applicable copyright law. Any unauthorized distribution or use of this text may be a direct infringement of the author s and publisher s rights and those responsible may be liable in law accordingly.

Imprint:

Copyright © 2016 GRIN Verlag, Open Publishing GmbH
Print and binding: Books on Demand GmbH, Norderstedt Germany
ISBN: 9783668350526

This book at GRIN:

http://www.grin.com/en/e-book/344711/the-main-principles-for-the-management-of-health-organizations

Bruce Wembulua

The main principles for the management of health organizations

GRIN Publishing

GRIN - Your knowledge has value

Since its foundation in 1998, GRIN has specialized in publishing academic texts by students, college teachers and other academics as e-book and printed book. The website www.grin.com is an ideal platform for presenting term papers, final papers, scientific essays, dissertations and specialist books.

Visit us on the internet:

http://www.grin.com/

http://www.facebook.com/grincom

http://www.twitter.com/grin_com

The main principles for the management of health organizations.

Dr WEMBULUA SHINGA BRUCE

Student of online Master of Science in Health Management

UNIVERSITÀ TELEMATICA INTERNAZIONALE UNINETTUNO.

This piece of work describe succinctly the main principles of health management as applied in the actual modern context.

Academic year 2016 -2017

INTRODUCTION

It is known that better health leads to faster economic growth which in turn, catalyzed by the equitable distribution of wealth, leads to healthier populations (Kovacic and Lijana 2008:3). Given this statement, the introduction of management notions in health care provision can be considered as one of the more relevant health sector innovations of our era.

Management has been discussed, practiced, and written about since the beginning of time. Although health care management as a separate discipline is of more recent origin (Healey and Marchese 2012: 10), it is sustained by solid principles stated a long before by famous theorists such as Frederick Taylor, father of scientific management, Henri Fayol - who developed "Fayolism"-, Max Weber and many others. Most of them asserted that health care management, as part of management in general, involves certain functions and activities that must be performed to achieve effectively and efficiently the set goals of the organization (Healey and Marchese 2012).

As there is continuous need to improve the quality of health services (Healey and Marchese 2012), improving the efficiency and effectiveness of health care provision will require well-developed skills among managers. These skills come through clear understanding of basic principles that sustain efficient application of management in health organizations. Lines below, try to describe succinctly main principles of health management as applied in the actual modern context.

CHAPTER 1: FUNDAMENTALS OF HEALTH MANAGEMENT

Management is the process of getting work done through others. As a process, Management consists of achieving organizational goals through planning, organizing, directing, and controlling human and physical resources (Swanwick and Mc Kimm 2011, Mokhlis 2011)

1. MANAGEMENT FUNCTIONS

There is enough disagreement among management writers on the classification of managerial functions. In the context of this work, we have considered Fayol's 5 functions which still form the basis of much of modern management thought and action (Tripathi and Reddy 2008).

   a. **Planning**

Planning involves those activities associated with objectives setting, policy making, and developing strategies for attaining objectives within the organizational policy framework. (Goldsmith 2011, Tripathi and Reddy 2008).

   b. **Organizing**

To organize a business is to provide it with everything useful to its functioning: personnel, raw materials, tools, capital - all designed as human and material resources. (Tripathi and Reddy 2008).

   c. **Commanding and Coordinating**

In carrying out these functions the Manager explains to his people what they have to do and helps them to do it to the best of their ability. He uses his position to guide, to persuade, or to coach subordinates. So this function includes three sub-functions: **Communication, Leadership** and **Motivation** (Goldsmith 2011, Tripathi and Reddy 2008).

   d. **Controlling**

Controlling is concerned with the measurement of the performance against some predetermined standard. The Manager must ensure that everything occurs in conformity with the plan adopted, the instructions issued and the principles established. (Tripathi and Reddy 2008).

It is very importance to emphasize that the controlling function is an ongoing process taking place throughout the plan execution, not at its end.

All of these functions take place on an ongoing basis, realizing what Luka Kovacic identified as "The Management cycle" as depicted on the Figure 1 below.

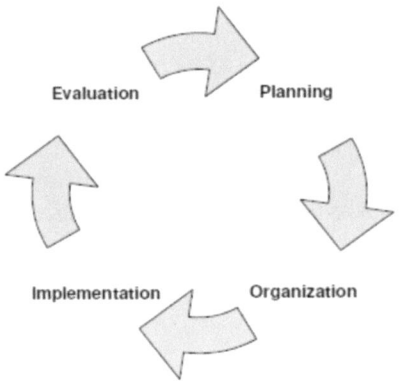

Fig 1. Management cycle: From planning to evaluation (Kovacic and Lijana 2008:4)

2. LEVELS OF MANAGEMENT

In any organization we found three main managerial levels:

- Lower (Fist-line) management: Made up of foremen or supervisors. They are in charge of direct coordination of functioning units of the organization.
- Top management: coordinates all the specialties and make policies for the company as a whole.
- Middle management: This level maintain communicative link between the top and lower management.

3. MANAGERIAL SKILLS

The management skills are required to carry out various functions of management. Three different types of skills are identified: Technical skills (First line managers), Human skills (Managers at all levels), and conceptual skills (particularly important for the top managers).

4. STRATEGIC MANAGEMENT

The health care industry is one of the most dynamic sectors. Successful health care organizations are those that have leaders who understand the nature and implications of external change, the ability to develop effective strategies that account for change, and the will as well as the ability to actively manage the momentum of the organization. These activities are collectively referred to as "strategic management. (Ginter, Duncan and Swayne 2013, Healey and Marchese 2012). To be effective, strategic management entails a clearly defined sense of purpose, which is captured in a mission statement and reflected in the goals and strategies set by the organization. (Healey and Marchese 2012).

CHAPTER 2: THEORIES AND PRINCIPLES OF HEALTH MANAGEMENT

1. CLASSICAL VIEWPOINT OF MANAGEMENT

Classical viewpoint covers early works and contributions that are the roots of the management (Bagad 2007).

1.1 Scientific management

The theory of scientific management was developed by Frederick Taylor. Taylor's theory required scientific selection of workers for job, managers' cooperation with workers, and the division of the work equally among workers and managers. (Healey and Marchese 2012, Tripathi and Reddy 2008, Bagad 2007). We can see that this principle finds a prior place in the hospital management since medical issues have to do with a delicate matter: the human life. So, objective selection of workers as well as clear definition and effective managerial coordination of tasks assigned are crucial. Positive cooperation between management and workers in the context of a hospital dispels frustration and promotes an effective workspace for the patients' welfare.

1.2 Administrative management

Henri Fayol is considered the Father of Administrative Management theory (Healey and Marchese 2012). The Fayol's theory focuses on the development of board administrative principles (Described below) applicable to general and higher managerial levels (Tripathi and Reddy 2008). Up to Fayol's principle, every enterprise desirous to be successful has to function as a single unit. This requires a clear established chain of command putting special stress on discipline, order and the will to comply first with the common interest.

1.3 Bureaucracy

This approach of management was developed by Max Weber. According to Weber, rules and regulations, along with a very clear hierarchy of authority, need to be present in a business to defeat the competition (Healey and Marchese 2012, Tripathi and Reddy 2008). In the actual context of health care characterized by continuous change, this principle can be effective if the established hierarchy is simple (clearly defined and understood) and flexible. This to dispel confusion so as to create a compatible workspace to innovative changes.

2. HENRI FAYOL'S PRINCIPLES OF MANAGEMENT (Tripathi and Reddy 2008, Bagad 2007, Anbuvelan, K. 2007).

Fayol outlined a number of principles that he found useful in running his large organization.

1. Division of Work

Division of work or work specialization results in efficient use of resources and increase productivity. In practice, employees are specialized in different areas and they have different skills. Therefore, continuous thinking of how to subdivide the hospital in more specialized functioning units will increase both the quality of service and productivity.

2. **Authority and Responsibility**

In order to get things done in an organization, management has the authority to give orders to the employees. Of course with this authority comes responsibility which cannot be shared with subordinates.

3. **Discipline**

Discipline means following rules, regulations, policies and procedures by all employees of organization. There must be clear and fair agreement for observing rules and regulations also punishment for disobedience and indiscipline. This management principle is essential and is seen as the oil to make the engine of an organization run smoothly.

4. **Unity of Command**

The management principle 'Unity of command' means that an individual employee should receive orders from one manager and that the employee is answerable to that manager to avoid confusion which may lead to possible conflicts for employees.

5. **Unity of Direction**

All the activities must be aimed at one common objective. The activities should be organized such that there should be one plan and one person in charge. This enables direction of efforts towards attainment of one goal.

6. **Subordination of Individual Interest**

In order to have an organization function well, Henri Fayol indicated that personal interests should be subordinate to the interests of the organization (ethics). The primary focus is on the organizational objectives and not on those of the individual. That why the modern heath service provision is "patient centered". All the organization works for the patients' health promotion.

7. **Remuneration**

The remuneration (non-monetary or monetary) should be sufficient to keep employees motivated and productive. This is particularly important in health sectors considering the highly need for accuracy. So employees should be well and continuously highly motivated.

8. **The Degree of Centralization**

The centralization of authority and power to some extent is necessary where it is most feasible otherwise there should be decentralization for smooth functioning of the organization. A balance between both must be achieved.

9. **Scalar Chain**

Henri Fayol's "hierarchy" management principle states that there should be a clear line in the area of authority (from top to bottom and all managers at all levels). Each employee can contact a manager or a superior in an emergency situation without challenging the hierarchy.

10. **Order**

Order is principle of arrangement of things and people. Everything should occupy its proper place and the right person in the right place. Order is the cornerstone principle for a hospital to act efficiently especially in case of emergencies so as to avoid fatal mistakes (transmission of diseases, confusion between vials, etc.)

11. **Equity**

According to Henri Fayol, employees must be treated kindly and equally. Organization is run better when managers are fair with their employees. There is no place for friction or frustration in a health care workspace since this can anytime cost a human life. So equity is more than important in such sectors.

12. **Stability of Personnel Tenure**

Management should strive to minimize employee turnover and to have the right staff in the right place because time is required to become effective in new jobs. This principle must be taken into account in the context of the hospital. Wondering from a department to another reduce the quality of service.

13. Initiative

Managers should encourage and develop the subordinates to take initiative. It is the result of creative thinking and imagination. This principle is possible only if employees are given the chance to do so through a propitious environment. The fear of punishment can simply collapse any tendency to think innovatively.

14. Esprit de Corps

Since union is strength, harmony and team work are essential in any organization.

CONCLUSIONS

Management refers to getting work done through others. It is the process of achieving goals through planning, organizing, directing, and controlling available resources at each managerial level within an organization. Taking into account the continuous environment change, each organization should consider strategic management to provide effective and efficient services.

Taken either as a science or an art, management has been discussed, practiced, and written about since the beginning of time. That why the current modern approach of management has its foundation laid on principles stated a long before by famous theorists such as Frederick Taylor, Henri Fayol, Max Weber and others.

Many of the principles stated by these authors are still of great importance in the current modern health organizations. Given the need for accuracy within the hospital, staffing and scientific definition of tasks assigned must take into account the scientific approach of Taylor. A simple, clear and flexible chain of command should be established within the organization to effectively cope with crisis and change by acting as a single unit putting special stress to comply first with the common interest.

As the health sector is more sensible, it is reasonable to keep the employees' moral higher through correct and continuous motivation. Discipline toward protocols and policies settled, order which allows everyone and everything to be in a right place, facilitate smooth functioning of the organization and minimizes mistakes that should be avoided as firmly as possible.

BIBLIOGRAPHY

1. Anbuvelan, K. (2007). *Principles of Management.* New Delhi, Laxmi Publications LTD.
2. Bagad V.S. (2007). *Principles of Management.* India, Technical publication Pune.
3. Ginter P. M., Duncan J., Swayne E.L. (2013). *The Strategic Management of Health Care Organizations.* 7th ed. England, John Wiley & sons Ltd.
4. Goldsmith, S. B. (2011). *Principles of Health Care Management: Foundations for a Changing Health Care System.* 2d ed. London, Jones and Bartlett Publishers, LLC.
5. Healey, B. and Marchese, M. (2012). *Foundations of Health Care Management: Principles and Methods.* San Francisco, John Wiley & Sons, Inc.
6. Kovacic, L. and Lijana, Z-K. (2008). *Management in health care practice: A handbook for teachers, Researchers and Health Professionals.* Zagreb, Hans Jacobs publishing company.
7. Mokhlis, A. (2011). *Principles of Health Management.* [online] available from https://medicalphys.files.wordpress.com/2011/03/lecture-1.ppt [12-9-2016].
8. Swanwick, T., Mc Kimm, J. (2011). *ABC of clinical Leadership.* Oxford, Wiley-Blackwell.
9. Tripathi P.C., Reddy P.N. (2008). *Principles of Management.* 4th Ed. New Delhi, Tata McGraw-Hill Publishing Company limited.

YOUR KNOWLEDGE HAS VALUE

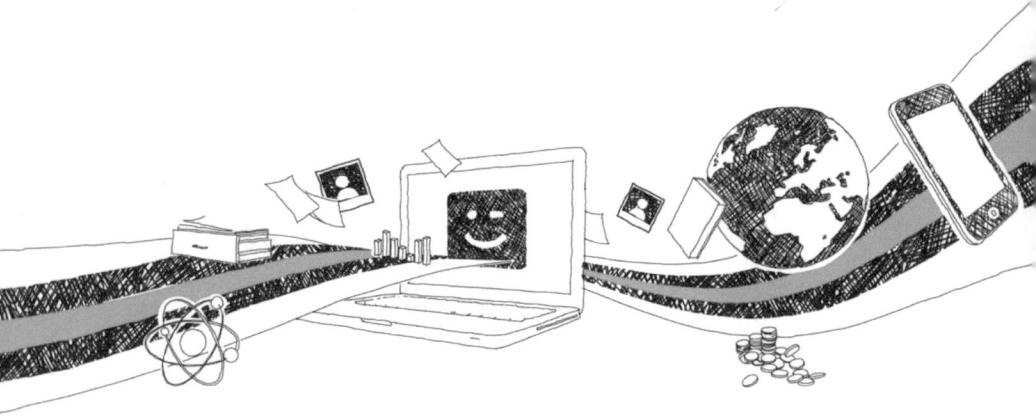

- We will publish your bachelor's and master's thesis, essays and papers

- Your own eBook and book - sold worldwide in all relevant shops

- Earn money with each sale

Upload your text at www.GRIN.com and publish for free

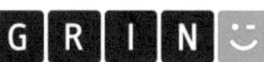